HOMŒOPATHY FOR YOUR PETS

An Introduction to the use
of classical homœopathic medicines
in the treatment of common
ailments in domestic animals

Recommended by
HOMŒOPATHIC DEVELOPMENT FOUNDATION LTD

CONTENTS

INTRODUCTION

For many years homœopathic medicines have been recognised as a safe and effective way of treating illness - in humans and in animals. Homœopathy for animals was in widespread use in the nineteenth and early twentieth centuries. Now in the twenty-first century we are rediscovering the value of homœopathy for pets.

Homœopathic remedies are ideal to use in the relief of symptoms of all diseases and conditions of pets. Modern homœopathic pharmacies produce remedies to an impeccable standard of quality, using pure natural sources. Remedies are safe to use, when given as directed. The use of homœopathic medicine may mean that conventional drugs will not be required; but homœopathy can also be used as a complementary therapy for patients that need conventional medication.

It is important to remember that this booklet is not a substitute for veterinary treatment. The remedies suggested will undoubtedly be of help to your pet. However, any symptoms of serious illness, or any symptoms which persist for more than a few days must have veterinary attention as soon as possible. Never continue with homœopathic medicines if your pet's condition is getting worse.

On the following pages you will find an explanation of what homœopathy is, how it began, how it can help animals, how to select the correct remedy for your pet, and how to administer and store remedies. Please make sure you read the information on choosing remedies and on dose rates before you begin to use homœopathic medicines for your pet.

Homœopathy is a gentle, safe and effective method of treatment. Your pet will thank you for choosing to use homœopathy!

WHAT IS HOMŒOPATHY?

The name homœopathy comes from the Greek word homeo, meaning 'like', and pathos, meaning 'suffering'. The principle of homœopathy can be summed up as 'like treats like'. In other words, a substance which causes certain symptoms when taken as a material dose, can be used to cure those symptoms when given to a patient with disease.

For instance homœopathic Arsenic is used to treat gastro-enteritis and food poisoning, the symptoms of which are exactly the same as those caused by taking the actual substance Arsenic. Or the homœopathic remedy Allium cepa (made from onions) is used to treat symptoms of hay fever - watery eyes, runny nose - exactly the symptoms caused when you chop an onion.

Homœopathic remedies act at a deep level in the body, and stimulate the body's own healing mechanisms. This is unlike conventional drugs such as steroids, which tend to suppress symptoms.

Homœopathy takes account of the whole patient, and not just the part of the body affected by disease, so homœopathy is a true holistic therapy. In homœopathic treatment, different patients with the same disease may need different remedies - because their individual symptoms will vary.

So, in essence, homœopathy is a way of stimulating the body's own healing processes, by using minute doses of substances that would normally cause the symptoms shown.

HOW DID HOMŒOPATHY BEGIN?

The principle of 'like treats like' has been known since the time of Hippocrates, the Greek 'father' of medicine, about 450 BC. A thousand years later the Swiss healer Paracelsus used the same principle of medicine, but it was not until the late 18th century that homœopathy as a fully investigated and validated system of medicine was developed.

The German physician and scholar Samuel Hahnemann was the originator of modern homœopathy. Horrified by the barbaric medical practice of his time, he developed homœopathy as a safe, gentle, effective alternative.

4

Hahnemann's first venture into homœopathy was his discovery that by taking small doses of cinchona bark (quinine), he developed mild symptoms of malaria. However, patients suffering from malaria could be cured by giving them doses of cinchona. The quinine seemed to trigger a reflex in the body which helped it cure itself.

Hahnemann experimented with various vegetable, animal and mineral substances and eventually catalogued over 200 useful remedies. All of these were "proved" by Hahnemann and his colleagues as substances which could both produce symptoms in healthy individuals, and cure the same symptoms in patients.

The next step was to find the smallest effective dose, to reduce the risk of side effects. Surprisingly, Hahnemann found that the more the remedy was diluted, the more effective it became in curing symptoms.

So Hahnemann found as he continued his work:

- a substance that in a large dose causes symptoms of disease will, in very small doses, cure those symptoms

- with extreme dilution, the curative properties increase, and all danger of toxic side effects are lost

- remedies should be prescribed by looking at the whole patient - not just their physical symptoms, but their character and temperament.

TREATING ANIMALS WITH HOMŒOPATHY

Animals respond well to homœopathy. From horses to hamsters, from Chihuahuas to chinchillas, whether with fur, feathers or scales, homœopathic treatments are effective. They are safe to use for puppies and kittens, for old animals, for pregnant pets. At any time of life, for any condition, homœopathy is an ideal therapy. Its use in animals rules out the 'placebo' effect - animals can't believe or imagine they are going to get better, so any effect is a real effect.

Because homœopathy relies on a close observation of symptoms, and takes into account the character, temperament, habits and preferences of the patient, it is important to know your pet well. Does your dog have a fear of thunder? Or a passion for chocolate? Does your cat always choose the warmest possible place to sleep? Is that itching nose in the evening, or in the morning, or at night? Does that ear infection always recur in one ear rather than the other? All such information is important when choosing the correct medication.

If you know your pets well, and watch them closely, you can treat minor problems with homœopathy rapidly and effectively, using the remedies listed in the following pages.

QUESTIONS AND ANSWERS

1. Is homœopathy safe?

Homœopathy is one of the safest forms of OTC medicine available because the active ingredients are present in extremely low concentrations. Homœopathy is renowned as being safe, non toxic and non addictive and is prepared in laboratories licensed by the Department of Health to stringent standards of quality. Homœopathy, like many conventional tablets and pillules, has small amounts of lactose, seek advice from your veterinary surgeon if your pet has a lactose intolerance.

2. Is homœopathy effective?

Homœopathy is as effective for animals as it is for humans and has often been used successfully where other forms of medicine have failed. In more recent years medical journals have published positive reports of the results of scientific research into homœopathy. There is an increasing number of veterinary surgeons practising homœopathy in the United Kingdom. Addresses are available from the British Homœopathic Association in London or the British Association of Homœopathic Veterinary Surgeons.

3. Is homœopathy recognised officially?

Homœopathy was recognised by an Act of Parliament in 1948, as a safe alternative form of medical treatment. Homœopathy is practised by doctors who are fully qualified through conventional medical training and it is recognised by the General Medical Council.

4. What are homœopathic potencies?

The potency is the number of times the mother tincture has been diluted. For example, if one drop of mother tincture is added to 99 drops of diluent (water or alcohol) and succussed (vigorously shaken) this is known as 1c potency. If one drop of this is then diluted in the same way, the resulting solution is 2c potency. This dilution can be repeated many times until the desired potency is achieved. The most commonly used potencies are 6c and 30c.

5. How do I know which potency to use?

The principles of homœopathy mean that the more dilute a remedy, the more potent it becomes. As a general rule, for most acute and long-standing ailments, the 6c potency is most suitable. In emergencies and in many chronic conditions, 30c remedies are better. However, it is more important to select the correct remedy than to use the right potency.

6. What reactions can I expect when using homœopathic remedies?

A slight increase in symptoms may be experienced at the start of treatment. These are known as 'aggravations' and are a sign that the body's own natural healing powers are starting to work. If this happens you should stop taking the remedies until the aggravation subsides and then restart. If the symptoms continue to worsen after stopping the remedy, it could be that the condition is worsening and you should seek advice from your veterinary surgeon.

7. What should I do if some symptoms improve but others don't or if new symptoms appear?

In this case, a second remedy should be started based on the remaining or new symptoms.

8. Does taking a larger dose have a greater effect?

No. It is the frequency of taking the dose that matters, not the number of tablets or pillules.

9. How should homœopathic medicines be stored?

All homœopathic medicines should be kept in their original container, away from direct light and strong smelling substances such as toothpaste, mint, perfume, aromatherapy oils, mothballs, menthol inhalants and rubefacients. If any tablets, pillules or granules are spilled they should not be returned to the container.

10. Can homœopathic medicines be taken with ordinary drugs?

It is safe to take homœopathy whilst taking allopathic medicines. However, any side-effects that are caused by the allopathic drug may complicate the symptom picture and make the correct choice of a homœopathic medicine more difficult. Always follow your veterinary surgeon's advice.

POPULAR HOMŒOPATHIC REMEDIES

There are several thousand homœopathic remedies available in a wide range of different potencies of which 6c and 30c potencies are the most common. The following is a list of homœopathic remedies that are stocked in most pharmacies and health food stores. Remedies that have not been included in the list are generally available either by mail order or from specialist homœopathic pharmacies.

1. Aconitum napellus **(Aconite)**
2. Apis mellifica **(Apis mel.)**
3. Argentum nitricum **(Argent. nit.)**
4. Arnica montana **(Arnica)**
5. Arsenicum album **(Arsen. alb.)**
6. Belladonna **(Belladonna)**
7. Bryonia dioica **(Bryonia)**
8. Calcarea carbonica **(Calc. carb.)**
9. Calcarea fluorica **(Calc. fluor.)**
10. Carbo vegetabilis **(Carbo veg.)**
11. Euphrasia officinalis **(Euphrasia)**
12. Gelsemium sempervirens **(Gelsemium)**
13. Graphites **(Graphites)**
14. Hepar sulphuris **(Hepar sulph.)**
15. Hypericum perforatum **(Hypericum)**
16. Ignatia amara **(Ignatia)**
17. Ipecacuanha **(Ipecac.)**
18. Kalium bichromicum **(Kali. bich.)**
19. Kalium phosphoricum **(Kali. phos.)**
20. Lycopodium clavatum **(Lycopodium)**
21. Mercurius solubilis **(Merc. sol.)**
22. Natrum muriaticum **(Nat. mur.)**
23. Nux vomica **(Nux vom.)**
24. Pulsatilla nigricans **(Pulsatilla)**
25. Rhus toxicodendron **(Rhus tox.)**
26. Ruta graveolens **(Ruta grav.)**
27. Sepia **(Sepia)**
28. Silicea **(Silicea)**
29. Sulphur **(Sulphur)**
30. Thuja occidentalis **(Thuja)**

Before giving any remedy, read the instructions on how to select, administer and store remedies, which follows.

SELECTING THE CORRECT HOMŒOPATHIC REMEDY

The remedy and disease guide which follows is in two parts.

The first part is a list of symptoms and diseases in alphabetical order. The second part is a list of homœopathic remedies and their action. By comparing the two lists, the appropriate remedy can be chosen.

Selecting the remedy:

1. Look up the symptoms from which your pet is suffering in the Index of Symptoms (pages 13 - 22)

2. Look at the descriptions of medicines and their actions.

3. Choose the remedy which most closely matches the symptoms shown and always get veterinary attention if symptoms persist or get worse.

Never treat acute problems on your own - always obtain veterinary treatment first. However, homœopathic remedies can be safely added to any conventional medicines.

Other Preparations

Apart from tablets, remedies are available as:

Ointments and Creams

Apply to affected area twice daily.

Tinctures

For external use: dilute by adding one drop of tincture to 10 drops of water. Apply to affected area twice daily.

For Eyes

Add 3 drops of tincture to 10 ml (2 tsps) of cooled, boiled water and bathe the eyes with this twice daily. Never put in the eyes undiluted.

HOW TO USE HOMŒOPATHIC REMEDIES

Selecting the potency

Remedies are produced in different strengths (potencies). This means that during the manufacturing process, the original substance is increasingly diluted to different strengths, which are called potencies. Remedies are available in many different potencies. In general it is best to use the 6c potency for pets.

How to administer

Ideally a remedy should be placed directly in the mouth, at least half an hour away from feeding time. Tablets can be crushed into a powder, if this is easier. For pets who dislike taking tablets (usually cats!) the tablet can be mixed with a small amount of butter, margarine, or bland food such as fish. Or tablets can be dissolved in a little milk or water. Do not give with a large amount of food, if possible. Preferably do not give any strong smelling or tasting substances, such as garlic, while homœopathic remedies are being administered. Do not handle tablets directly - use the cap of the container as a dispenser, or use containers with 'built in' dispensers.

Dosage and frequency

For acute problems, such as shock or haemorrhage, give one tablet every five minutes for up to one hour.

For severe, but less acute, symptoms, such as diarrhoea, give one tablet every fifteen minutes for three hours, then one hourly for the rest of the day. Then give one tablet three times daily for three days, or until symptoms have disappeared.

For chronic symptoms, such as persistent itchy skin, give one tablet three times daily for one week, followed by one tablet twice daily for two weeks.

In all cases stop giving remedies if the symptoms disappear completely.

Storage

Store remedies in a cool, dry place away from direct light, and away from any strong smelling substances such as mint, perfume, aromatherapy oils and mothballs. If any tablets, pillules or granules are spilled they should not be returned to the container.

Stored properly, remedies will remain active for many years.

Response to a homœopathic remedy

Sometimes the symptoms may become worse. Do not be alarmed as this indicates that the medicine is working. If this happens postpone the dose until this increase or 'aggravation' as it is known, has passed.

Side effects

Due to the extreme dilutions involved, there are no known side effects or contraindications to homœopathy. However, because small doses of lactose are used in the formulation of homœopathic tablets, granules and pillules, seek advice from your veterinary surgeon if your pet has a lactose intolerance.

Interactions

There are no known interactions between homœopathic remedies and other medicines, so it is acceptable to recommend a homœopathic remedy alongside a conventional treatment.

As with everything, practice and familiarity are the key. The better you get to know the remedies and their reactions the more accurate your selection will be and therefore the more effective the remedies will become.

INDEX OF SYMPTOMS

SYMPTOM	DESCRIPTION	REMEDY
Abdomen	Discomfort after overeating	*Nux vom.*
	Bloating with audible rumbling	*Carbo veg.*
	Pain and bloating after eating small amounts	*Lycopodium*
Abrasions	For unbroken skin	*Arnica*
	For broken skin (externally use Calendula and Hypericum tincture solution).	*Hypericum*
Abscess	Acute, with inflammation, painful when touched	*Hepar sulph.*
	Chronic, persistent	*Silicea*
	Mouth abscesses	*Merc. sol.*
Aggression	Aggressive behaviour	*Belladonna*
Allergies	Skin allergy with swollen, shiny skin	*Apis mel.*
	Skin allergy with hot itchy skin	*Sulphur*
Alopecia (fur loss)	In chilly animals who need warmth	*Arsen. alb.*
	Where the skin is also dry and cracked	*Nat. mur.*
Anaemia	For a tendency to be always anaemic	*Silicea*
	Anaemia with digestive problems	*Arsen. alb.*
	Anaemia with weakness and fever	*Ferr. phos*
Anal Glands	For acute inflammation with abscesses (also apply Calendula Cream)	*Hepar sulph.*
Appetite	Lack of (for simple digestive upsets)	*Carbo veg.*
	Lack of (with constipation)	*Nux vom.*
	Animal appears to want food but rejects it	*Arsen. alb.*
	Eats unusual things such as soil, or eats faeces	*Calc. carb.*
Arthritis	Worse for first movement after rest, but better for continued exercise	*Rhus. tox.*
	With much swelling	*Apis mel.*

SYMPTOM	DESCRIPTION	REMEDY
Arthritis (contd)	If the joints are bruised	*Arnica*
	With bone disease	*Calc. fluor.*
	Better at rest, but worse for movement	*Bryonia*
Bad Breath	Due to decayed or weak teeth	*Calc. fluor.*
	Due to accumulation of tartar and sore gums	*Merc. sol.*
	Due to gastric upsets	*Carbo veg.*
	With constipation	*Nux vom.*
	Following stress	*Kali. phos.*
Balanitis (inflammation of the penis with discharge)	Yellow or green discharge	*Merc. sol.*
	Creamy, profuse discharge	*Pulsatilla*
	(externally use Calendula and Hypericum tincture solution)	
Bereavement	Loss of litter, loss of companion	*Ignatia*
Biliousness	After eating	*Nux vom.*
	With kidney disease	*Apis mel.*
	With liver disease and jaundice	*Merc. sol.*
Bites (see also insect bites)	Punctured	*Hypericum*
	(externally use Calendula and Hypericum tincture solution)	
Bleeding gums	With bad breath	*Merc. sol.*
Blinking	Frequent, often with discharge from the eyes	*Euphrasia*
Breath	See *Bad Breath*	
Bruises	Superficial	*Arnica*
	Deeper bruises	*Ruta grav.*

SYMPTOM	DESCRIPTION	REMEDY
Burns	Most cases	*Burn cream*
	For accompanying shock	*Aconite*
Canker	See *Ear Infections*	
Cataracts	To help slow down development of	*Calc. fluor.*
Chorea	Nervous trembling and twitching	*Arsen. alb.*
Colic	For acute cases	*Nux vom.*
	With flatulence	*Argent. nit.*
Conjunctivitis	Simple, uncomplicated	*Argent. nit.*
	With creamy discharge	*Pulsatilla*
	After travelling with the head out of the car window	*Aconite*
	Where the margins of lids are red	*Euphrasia*
Constipation	Simple, uncomplicated	*Carbo veg.*
	With loss of appetite	*Nux vom.*
	With skin disease	*Sulphur*
	During pregnancy	*Sepia*
	Small hard stools, difficult to pass	*Lycopodium*
Convulsions	With fever	*Belladonna*
	From stress	*Ignatia*
	From teething	*Chamomilla Granules*
Coprophagia (eating own faeces)	In overweight pets that scavenge	*Calc. carb.*
Cough	Dry cough, better at rest	*Bryonia*
	Spasmodic	*Ipecac.*
	Deep cough, with flaring nostrils	*Lycopodium*
Cracks/Fissures	Especially in the folds of the limbs	*Graphites*

SYMPTOM	DESCRIPTION	REMEDY
Cuts	Bathe with Calendula and Hypericum tincture solution or use Calendula Cream	
Cystitis	With high temperature	*Belladonna*
	With difficulty in passing urine	*Apis mel.*
	With straining, red sediment in urine	*Lycopodium*
Dandruff	With dry, scaly skin	*Arsen. alb.*
	With hot, itchy skin	*Sulphur*
Dermatitis	See *Eczema*	
Diarrhoea	With watery stools	*Arsen. alb.*
	With slimy, blood-stained stools	*Merc. sol.*
	In nervous animals	*Argent. nit.*
	With vomiting	*Arsen. alb., Ipecac.*
Distress	See *Shock*	
Dysentery	Slimy stools, worse at night	*Merc. sol.*
	For accompanying vomiting	*Ipecac.*
	See also *Diarrhoea, Enteritis, Gastritis*	
Ear Infections	When acutely inflamed and sensitive to touch	*Hepar sulph.*
	Surface of ears scaly, with scabby edges	*Kali. bich.*
	Suppurating with evil smelling discharge	*Merc. sol.*
	Associated with dry skin and watery discharge, often worse late at night	*Arsen. alb.*
	Persistent cases	*Rhus tox.*
	Thick, yellow, offensive discharge	*Lycopodium*
Eczema	For pets preferring cool places, with hot, red skin	*Sulphur*
	For pets preferring warmth, with dry, scaly skin	*Arsen. alb.*
	For dry, cracked skins	*Nat. mur.*
	For sticky discharges	*Graphites*
	For violent itching, with skin fissures and ulceration	*Lycopodium*
Enteritis	Simple, uncomplicated cases	*Arsen. alb.*

16

SYMPTOM	DESCRIPTION	REMEDY
Epilepsy	In nervous animals	*Ignatia*
Exhaustion	After sickness Following stress	*Arnica* *Kali. phos.*
Eyelids	Inflamed, symptoms worsen after waking Swollen, with a yellow stringy discharge Ulceration and redness	*Rhus tox.* *Kali. bich.* *Lycopodium*
Eyes	Profuse watering from	*Euphrasia*
Fear	After a sudden shock Of noise, where sudden e.g. thunder and fireworks General hypersensitivity to noise	*Aconite* *Gelsemium* *Kali. phos.*
Fever	Very early stages Very high temperature and thirsty	*Aconite* *Belladonna*
Fireworks	Rigid with fear and anxiety	*Gelsemium*
Flatulence	Most cases Due to eating unsuitable food Caused by liver disease	*Carbo veg.* *Nux vom.* *Lycopodium*
Fractures	For fractures, dislocations and bone injuries	*Ruta grav.*
Gastritis	With accompanying diarrhoea With repeated vomiting	*Arsen. alb.* *Ipecac.*
Gums	Spongy and sore Swollen and tender	*Merc. sol.* *Apis mel.*
Hairball	To help animals (usually cats) either to vomit, or pass it	 *Nux vom.*
Hay fever	Watering eyes	*Euphrasia*
Heart conditions	With fluid congestion	*Apis mel.*

SYMPTOM	DESCRIPTION	REMEDY
Heat stroke	With great thirst	*Belladonna*
Hepatitis	See *Liver*	
Hiccough	In young puppies	*Ignatia*
	In very nervous animals	*Gelsemium*
Homesickness	For example, in boarding kennels	*Ignatia*
Horse-fly bites	To help reduce swelling	*Hypericum*
Hysteria	Accompanied by fits	*Belladonna*
Incontinence	In excitable young pets	*Ignatia*
(of urine)	In older animals	*Calc. fluor.*
Infections	With pus and discharge	*Hepar sulph.*
	With fever	*Belladonna*
	To help convalesce after	*Kali. phos.*
Inflammation	See *Ears, Penis, Anal Glands, Kidneys, Testicles*	
Injuries	With bruising	*Arnica*
	Involving nerves	*Hypericum*
	Sprains and strains	*Ruta grav.*
Insect bites	Wasps or bees	*Apis mel.*
	Horse-fly bites	*Hypericum*
	(Externally use Pyrethrum tincture solution)	
Insomnia		
(sleeplessness)	In older animals	*Arsen. alb.*
Jaundice	With vomiting and diarrhoea	*Merc. sol.*
Kidneys		
(Inflammation of)	See *Nephritis*	

18

SYMPTOM	DESCRIPTION	REMEDY
Liver disease	Caused by unsuitable food	**Nux vom.**
	With jaundice	**Merc. sol.**
	Hepatitis, with fever	**Belladonna**
	Chronic liver disease, often with fluid in the abdomen	**Lycopodium**
Mange	For pets who dislike heat	**Sulphur**
	For pets who prefer warmth	**Arsen. alb.**
Mastitis	For hot, painful glands	**Belladonna**
	Where glands feel hard	**Bryonia**
	For chronic, persistent mastitis	**Calc. fluor.**
Muscles	Weakness of	**Gelsemium**
Nasal discharge	Yellow stringy catarrh	**Kali. bich.**
	Creamy mucoid catarrh	**Pulsatilla**
	Watery sneezing	**Nat. mur.**
Nephritis (inflammation of the kidney)	Very acute with swelling of kidneys	**Apis mel.**
	Where associated with vomiting and skin disease	**Arsen. alb.**
	When very thirsty, with pale coloured urine	**Nat. mur.**
Nipples	Cracked and sore (also apply Calendula Cream)	**Graphites**
Noise	General hypersensitivity	**Kali. phos.**
Nose bleeds (epistaxic)	Bright red blood, with vomiting	**Ipecac.**
	Bright red blood, with sneezing	**Aconite**
Operations	To aid convalescence	**Kali. phos.**
	For constipation after operation	**Nux vom.**
	To minimise bruising	**Arnica**
Orchitis (inflammation of the testicles)	With extreme sensitivity to touch	**Hepar sulph.**
	Where fluid is present beneath the skin (dents remain in skin if pressure is applied)	**Apis mel.**

SYMPTOM	DESCRIPTION	REMEDY
Paralysis	Gradual onset	*Gelsemium*
	With nerve damage	*Hypericum*
Penis (inflammation of)	See *Balanitis*	
Pregnancy, false	Where the bitch is moody or vicious	*Sepia*
	With much milk	*Pulsatilla*
Pyometritis	With creamy discharge	*Pulsatilla*
	With fear and increased thirst	*Belladonna*
Restlessness	With frequent change of position	*Arsen. alb.*
Rheumatism	Where animal improves on exercise	*Rhus tox.*
	Where animal prefers to rest	*Bryonia*
	For acute conditions, sprains and strains	*Ruta grav.*
	In older, overweight animals	*Calc. carb.*
Ringworm	With circular patches, more on body than on head	*Sepia*
Seborrhoea	Dry, greasy skin	*Nat. mur.*
	Sticky and discharging skin	*Graphites*
Shock	Immediately afterwards	*Aconite*
	Followed by	*Arnica*
Show animals	Fright during show	*Gelsemium*
Skin Conditions	See *Eczema*	
Slipped Disc	For the pain	*Hypericum*
	For the stiffness	*Rhus tox.*
Sore throat	Painful and hot	*Belladonna*
	With tonsillitis, starting on right side	*Lycopodium*

SYMPTOM	DESCRIPTION	REMEDY
Sprains	Worse for rest, better for movement	*Rhus tox.*
	Combine with	*Ruta grav.*
Stiffness	Following exercise	*Arnica*
	Worse for rest, better for movement	*Rhus tox., Ruta grav.*
	Better for rest	*Bryonia*
Stings	See *Insect Bites*	
Strains	Worse at rest, better for movement	*Rhus tox.*
Swelling	Containing fluid	*Apis mel.*
Teething	Pain and discomfort	*Chamomilla Granules*
	When difficult and delayed	*Calc. carb.*
Testicles (inflammation of)	See *Orchitis*	
Thunder	'Rigid with fear'	*Gelsemium*
Tongue	Yellow coated	*Bryonia*
	Dry, following stress	*Kali. phos.*
Travel Sickness	With restlessness and fear	*Aconite*
	With vomiting	*Ipecac.*
Trembling, muscular	In old animals	*Kali. phos.*
	After too much exercise	*Rhus tox.*
Twitching	Muscular	*Belladonna*
	With restlessness	*Arsen. alb.*
Ulcers	In the mouth	*Merc. sol.*

SYMPTOM	DESCRIPTION	REMEDY
Uterus *(discharge)*	See *Pyometritis*	
Vaccinations	Adverse reaction to	*Thuja*
Vomiting	Accompanied by diarrhoea Spasmodic In thirsty animals	*Arsen. alb.* *Ipecac.* *Merc. sol.*
Warts	On any parts of body	*Thuja*
Wounds	See *Abrasions, Bites, Bruises, Cuts*	

THE MEDICINES AND THEIR INDICATIONS

MEDICINE/AILMENT OR CONDITION

REMARKS

1. Aconite (Aconitum napellus)

A remedy for fevers and inflammatory states
Complaints caused by exposure to cold dry winds
Complaints caused by severe fright
Shivering with cold sweats
Breathing difficult
Upper part of body hot while the lower body cold
Animal wants large amounts of water
Acute anxiety
Travel sickness
Restlessness

Symptoms worse:
around midnight
in a warm room
in cold winds

Symptoms better:
in the open air

2. Apis mel. (Apis mellifica)

A remedy for inflammation or injury
Swellings containing fluid
Arthritis and swelling
Swollen gums
Biliousness
Insect bites
Inflammation of testicles
Animal seeks cold surface to lie on

Symptoms worse:
from heat
when touched
in closed and heated rooms
after sleeping

Symptoms better:
for cold bathing
in the open air

3. Argent. nit. (Argent nitricum)

Nervous animal with trembling
Diarrhoea
Colic
Much flatulence
Conjunctivitis
Weakness in limbs

Symptoms worse:
with warmth
at night

MEDICINE/AILMENT OR CONDITION

REMARKS

4. Arnica (Arnica montana)

A remedy for accidents and injury
Use after an injury
To lessen shock
Bruises
Sprains
Exhaustion after over-exercise
After dental extraction
The animal shrinks away from touch

Symptoms worse:
from touch
from movement
in damp, cold conditions

Symptoms better:
when lying down

5. Arsen. alb. (Arsenicum album)

A remedy where the animal will show much
fear and restlessness
Animal shows no interest in food
Alopecia (loss of fur)
Chilly animals who love warmth
Temperature normal but gums and lips may be cold
Insomnia in older animals
Anaemia
Dandruff
Ear infections
Eczema
Enteritis
Gastritis
Mange

Symptoms worse:
after midnight
in cold wet weather

Symptoms better:
for warmth

6. Belladonna (tropa belladonna)

A main fever remedy
Fever with heat, redness, pain and swelling
Aggressive behaviour
Convulsion
Hysteria which sometimes leads to fits
Mastitis
Muscular twitching
Inflammation in the ear
Heat stroke

Symptoms worse:
from noise
from touch
from lying down

Symptoms better:
for quietness and
in the dark

MEDICINE/AILMENT OR CONDITION	REMARKS

7. *Bryonia (Bryonia alba)*

Dry mouth

Great thirst

Yellow coated tongue

Arthritis

Rheumatism

Cough

Mastitis

Animal prefers to lie still since movement increases its discomfort

Animal also prefers to lie on affected part as pressure relieves symptoms

Symptoms worse:
from any movement

8. *Calc. carb. (Calcarea carbonica)*

A remedy for overweight sluggish animals

Bone disorder in fat young animals

Very fat puppies

Teething delayed

Conjunctivitis

Excessive appetite

Symptoms worse:
from cold
in damp weather
at night

Symptoms better:
in dry weather
for warmth while lying
on affected part

9. *Calc. fluor. (Calcarea fluorica)*

Arthritis

Incontinence

Mastitis

Brittle bones

Poor teeth

Symptoms worse:
after rest
in damp weather

Symptoms better:
after a little movement
from warm applications

10. *Carbo. veg. (Carbo vegetabilis)*

Simple digestive upsets which cause loss of appetite

Bad breath

Constipation

Flatulence - frequent breaking of wind

Symptoms worse:
during warm damp weather
in the evening and at night
Symptoms better:
for passing wind
for cold

MEDICINE/AILMENT OR CONDITION	REMARKS

11. Euphrasia (Euphrasia officinalis)

A remedy for eye ailments

Watering eyes, often in dogs following a car journey with an open window

Conjunctivitis

Frequent blinking

Catarrhal discharge from the eyes

Hay fever

Symptoms worse:
in warm winds
when indoors
in smoky room

Symptoms better:
in dim light or darkness

12. Gelsemium (Gelsemium sempervirens)

Timid animals

Fright in show animals

Fear can cause animal to pass urine

Muscular weakness

Weak and trembling limbs

Symptoms worse:
from damp
from excitement

Symptoms better:
in the open air
after passing urine

13. Graphites (Graphites)

A remedy for skin conditions

Most commonly occurs in the folds of limbs or behind the ears, often with a sticky discharge

Eczema

Cracked and sore nipples

Cracks and fissures

Skin smells badly

Symptoms worse:
in cold and draughts

Symptoms better:
in the dark
from covering up,
and warmth

14. Hepar sulph. (Hepar sulphuris)

Characterised by extreme sensitivity to touch; the animal is often irritable

Particularly helpful in cases of suppuration

Any condition where pus has formed

Acute abscess with inflammation

Inflammation of the anal glands

Excessive thirst

Ear infection with inflammation

Inflammation of the testicles

Symptoms worse:
in cold air
when affected part
is touched
in draughts

Symptoms better:
in warm dry weather
in damp wet weather

MEDICINE/AILMENT OR CONDITION	REMARKS

15. *Hypericum (Hypericum perforatum)*

A remedy to help reduce pain
Especially useful where the part is rich in
nerves e.g. the tail
Abrasions with broken skin
Bites where the skin is punctured
Horse-Fly bites
This remedy when given as well as Calendula Cream
gives the double benefit of promoting
healing and reducing pain

Symptoms worse:
from cold and damp
in a closed room

Symptoms better:
in warm dry weather
in the open air

16. *Ignatia (Ignatia amara)*

A remedy for the pining or homesick animal
While the owner is away
While in boarding kennels
Give this remedy immediately when rescuing an
abandoned or ill-treated animal
Bereavement following loss of litter
Hiccough
Convulsions as a result of abandonment

Symptoms worse:
with loneliness

Symptoms better:
with company

17. *Ipecac. (Ipecacuanha)*

A remedy for vomiting
Gastritis with repeated vomiting
Dysentery
Travel sickness with vomiting
Diarrhoea with vomiting (seek veterinary advice)
Respiratory difficulties

Symptoms worse:
while lying down
periodically

Symptoms better:
with pressure

18. *Kali. bich. (Kalium bichromicum)*

A remedy for catarrhal symptoms
Yellow stringy discharge
Catarrhal discharge
Swollen eyelids
Raw or obstructed nose
Ear infections

Symptoms worse:
during hot weather
in the morning

Symptoms better:
during cold weather

27

MEDICINE/AILMENT OR CONDITION	REMARKS

19. *Kali. phos. (Kalium phosphoricum)*

A remedy for the animal which has undergone stress

Exhaustion

Extreme fear of noise

As an aid to convalescence following an operation

Muscular trembling in old animals

Bad breath

Dry tongue

Symptoms worse:
from noise

Symptoms better:
from warmth
after eating

20. *Lycopodium (Lycopodium clavatum)*

A remedy for digestive, respiratory,
liver and urinary problems

Bloating and flatulence

Irritating coughs

Liking for sweet tasting foods

Hates to be left alone

Eats small amounts of food at a time

May go grey prematurely

Symptoms worse:
from heat
on the right side
from 4pm to 8pm

Symptoms better:
for movement
for warm food or fluids
for cool air

21. *Merc. sol. (Mercurius solubilis)*

Jaundice

Biliousness during jaundice

Vomiting in thirsty animals

Dysentery with slimy stools

Diarrhoea with slimy blood-stained stools

Inflammation of the penis

Mouth ulcers

Mouth abscesses

Spongy gums

Ears which suppurate with a badly-smelling discharge

Ears with a greenish discharge

Symptoms worse:
at night
in a warm room

Symptoms better:
with rest

22. *Nat. mur. (Natrum muriaticum)*

A remedy for kidney complaints

Nephritis

Urine very pale in colour

Eczema with a dry cracked skin

Symptoms worse:
while lying down
in sunshine

MEDICINE/AILMENT OR CONDITION	REMARKS

Nat. mur. (contd)

| Alopecia | *Symptoms better:* |
| Animals with a scrawny lean appearance | in the open air |

23. Nux vom. (Nux vomica)

Hairball	*Symptoms worse:*
Poor appetite often accompanied by constipation	from cold
Digestive upsets	from movement
Bad breath	
Colic	*Symptoms better:*
Flatulence	from warmth
Bilious after feeding	in the evening
Hiccough in young puppies	

24. Pulsatilla (Pulsatilla nigricans)

A remedy which helps relieve female animal complaints	*Symptoms worse:*
Placid, 'shy' animals	in the evening
Symptoms tend to vary greatly	from heat
False pregnancy	sudden chilling when hot
Creamy discharges	
Little thirst	*Symptoms better:*
Conjunctivitis with catarrhal symptoms	in the open air
	after cold food and drink

25. Rhus tox. (Rhus toxicodendron)

A major rheumatic remedy	*Symptoms worse:*
Use this remedy if the animal's symptoms improve	with first movement
with a little exercise	after rest
Rheumatism	from cold and wet
Arthritis	during rest
Strains	
Sprains	*Symptoms better:*
Muscular trembling	after a little gentle exercise
Eyelids inflamed	during warm weather
Ear infections	

26. Ruta grav. (Ruta graveolens)

A main remedy for sprains or dislocations	*Symptoms worse:*
Acute rheumatism	from cold
Deep bruising	during wet weather

MEDICINE/AILMENT OR CONDITION	REMARKS

Ruta grav. (contd)
Injuries with resulting sprains
Fractures and bone injuries
Tendon and ligament injuries

Symptoms worse:
during rest

Symptoms better:
with warmth
with gentle exercise

27. Sepia (Sepia)
A remedy for the treatment of female
animal complaints
Unlike Pulsatilla the temperament is unpredictable
and can be vicious
False pregnancy
Animal is sensitive to cold
Constipation during pregnancy
Ringworm

Symptoms worse:
from cold
before thunder
in smoky rooms

Symptoms better:
with warmth
after gentle exercise
after rest

28. Silicea (Silicea)
A remedy to use when your animal has picked up a
splinter, thorn or other foreign body
Slow healing infections
Abscesses
Inflamed anal glands
Anaemia
Suited to animals which always retreat
should a fight start

Symptoms worse:
from cold
in cold weather
at the approach of winter

Symptoms better:
with warmth

29. Sulphur (Sulphur)
A remedy for use in skin conditions. The animal
seeks cool places in which to lie
Skin appears dirty and may show red patches where
the animal is seen to scratch frequently
Skin smells badly
Passes wind with offensive smell
Mange
Eczema

Symptoms worse:
with heat
at rest

Symptoms better:
in fresh air

MEDICINE/AILMENT OR CONDITION	REMARKS

Sulphur (contd)
Dandruff
Constipation

30. *Thuja (Thuja occidentalis)*

A remedy for warty growths

Symptoms worse:

The animal may refuse all food in the morning

in damp air

After vaccination, this remedy can relieve any ill-effects

May help when it is observed that the animal has never

Symptoms better:

been fully well since vaccination

in dry conditions

HOMŒOPATHIC CASE STUDIES

As examples of how homœopathic remedies are chosen and used, here are a few sample cases from a homœopathic veterinary's practice.

Jodie, 5 year old Springer Spaniel

Jodie suffered from false pregnancies after each season. She would become moody and irritable, didn't want to be stroked or cuddled, and didn't want to go out for walks, although when she was taken out, seemed to be happier for a while afterwards. SEPIA was successfully used to minimise the symptoms.

Cassie, 7 year old Cavalier King Charles Spaniel

Cassie also suffered from false pregnancies. She was a gentle, shy dog, who didn't become irritable, but seemed to feel up one day and down the next. She produced lots of milk, which made her uncomfortable. She only seemed happy out in the open air. PULSATILLA was chosen, and always relieved the symptoms.

These two cases show that the same condition may need different homœopathic remedies, depending on the symptoms shown.

Bernard, a 6 year old St Bernard

After a booster vaccination Bernard was unwell for a few days. He then developed an itchy skin, conjunctivitis with watery eyes, and spells of sickness and diarrhoea. Remedies such as SULPHUR and ARSEN. ALB. helped to some extent, but when THUJA was given, the symptoms disappeared completely.

This case shows that is can be important in homœopathy to look for the original cause of a problem, not just at the present symptoms.

Hoppy, a 2 year old rabbit

Hoppy had severe indigestion and colic after being left on his own in a shed containing a large bag of rabbit food. He nibbled his way through the bag and through most of its contents, and unsurprisingly felt severely ill afterwards. NUX VOM. saved the day and he was soon back to normal.

This case shows that smaller pets can be helped by homœopathy just as much as dogs and cats can.

Bruce, a 17 year old Siamese

After his long term companion, Forsyth, died, Bruce went into a decline and refused to eat. He stopped grooming himself, lost weight rapidly, and would continually prowl around the house, as if looking for his missing friend. IGNATIA gradually relieved the symptoms, and within a short while Bruce was back to his former self again.

This case shows how homœopathy can help emotional and behavioural, as well as physical, problems.

Ernest, a 3 year old cat

Ernest developed a cough, which his owner treated with homœopathy. She tried BRYONIA, because the cough was dry, then IPECAC. because the cough was spasmodic. She tried HEPAR SULPH. in case it was caused by an infection. She used HYPERICUM as Ernest seemed to be in pain. Finally she took Ernest to a vet who found he had a needle stuck in his throat.

This case shows how important it is to take your pet to a veterinary surgeon if symptoms don't clear up quickly!

RICHARD ALLPORT

NOTES

NOTES

NOTES